EDUCATION IN A COMPETITIVE AND GLOBALIZING WORLD

ASSESSMENT OF PROFESSIONAL PRACTICE: PERCEPTIONS AND PRINCIPLES

EDUCATION IN A COMPETITIVE AND GLOBALIZING WORLD

Additional books in this series can be found on Nova's website under the Series tab.

Additional E-books in this series can be found on Nova's website under the E-book tab.

EDUCATION IN A COMPETITIVE AND GLOBALIZING WORLD

ASSESSMENT OF PROFESSIONAL PRACTICE: PERCEPTIONS AND PRINCIPLES

MARGARET FISHER
TRACEY PROCTOR-CHILDS
LYNNE CALLAGHAN
ALISON STONE
KELLY SNELL
AND
LISA CRAIG

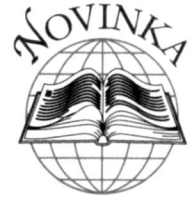

Nova Science Publishers, Inc.
New York

Copyright © 2011 by Nova Science Publishers, Inc.

All rights reserved. No part of this book may be reproduced, stored in a retrieval system or transmitted in any form or by any means: electronic, electrostatic, magnetic, tape, mechanical photocopying, recording or otherwise without the written permission of the Publisher.

For permission to use material from this book please contact us:
Telephone 631-231-7269; Fax 631-231-8175
Web Site: http://www.novapublishers.com

NOTICE TO THE READER

The Publisher has taken reasonable care in the preparation of this book, but makes no expressed or implied warranty of any kind and assumes no responsibility for any errors or omissions. No liability is assumed for incidental or consequential damages in connection with or arising out of information contained in this book. The Publisher shall not be liable for any special, consequential, or exemplary damages resulting, in whole or in part, from the readers' use of, or reliance upon, this material. Any parts of this book based on government reports are so indicated and copyright is claimed for those parts to the extent applicable to compilations of such works.

Independent verification should be sought for any data, advice or recommendations contained in this book. In addition, no responsibility is assumed by the publisher for any injury and/or damage to persons or property arising from any methods, products, instructions, ideas or otherwise contained in this publication.

This publication is designed to provide accurate and authoritative information with regard to the subject matter covered herein. It is sold with the clear understanding that the Publisher is not engaged in rendering legal or any other professional services. If legal or any other expert assistance is required, the services of a competent person should be sought. FROM A DECLARATION OF PARTICIPANTS JOINTLY ADOPTED BY A COMMITTEE OF THE AMERICAN BAR ASSOCIATION AND A COMMITTEE OF PUBLISHERS.

Additional color graphics may be available in the e-book version of this book.

LIBRARY OF CONGRESS CATALOGING-IN-PUBLICATION DATA
Assessment of professional practice : perceptions and principles / Margaret Fisher ... [et al.].
  p. cm.
 Includes bibliographical references.
 ISBN 978-1-61122-306-4 (softcover)
 1. Emergency medical personnel--Evaluation. 2. Midwives--Evaluation. 3. Social workers--Evaluation. I. Fisher, Margaret.
 RA645.5.A845 2010
 616.02'5092--dc22
                    2010037334

Published by Nova Science Publishers, Inc. † New York

CONTENTS

Preface		vii
Chapter 1	Introduction	1
Chapter 2	Methodology	5
Chapter 3	Findings	11
Chapter 4	Contextualising Our Research Study	39
Recommendations		45
Acknowledgments		49
References		51
Index		57

PREFACE

A multi-professional research team comprising practitioners, academics, service-users and students has undertaken a major research project on pre and post-registration students engaged in Social Work, Midwifery and Emergency Care (Nursing and Paramedicine) professional degrees. The aim of the study, under the auspices of the Centre for Excellence in Professional Placement Learning (Ceppl) at the University of Plymouth in the United Kingdom, has been to explore students' perceptions of the tools and methods used to assess their practice and the impact these processes have had on their learning and professionalism during their journey through the programme. A four-year longitudinal study comprising annual interviews with 14 students has enabled their developing understanding and changing views to emerge, rather than just gaining a snapshot as in previous literature. Single-case and cross-case analysis and synthesis using the Framework Technique has enabled individual, professional and cross-professional issues to be explored through the multiple case-study approach.

The main themes identified were: Process, Preparation, Purpose, Placements, People and Professional Persona – the six 'P's of practice assessment. Issues around reliability, validity, consistency, honesty, relationships with assessors and timing of suitable placements have been highlighted.

This book seeks to explain the methodology of the study and expound on the findings under the main themes. Comparisons are made between students' perceptions at the various stages of their programmes, and commonalities and differences between professional groups are explored. Principles of good practice are suggested in the 'Recommendations' chapter at the end which may be applied to a range of professional programmes incorporating placement learning and assessment.

Chapter 1

INTRODUCTION

The value of practice placements in any professional educational programme cannot be over-emphasised. This is particularly the case in health and social care professions. Through exposure to the real-life setting, students have the opportunity to develop the knowledge, skills and attributes essential to their role as practitioners of the future. As Cowburn, Nelson and Williams [2000] assert in their research in a Social Work context, the primary purpose of assessment is to safeguard people in receipt of such services. Therefore every effort should be made to ensure that assessment methods used are valid and reliable, enabling accurate judgement of the student's ability to practise safely and competently. A literature review undertaken by Chambers in 1998 identified problems in professional practice assessment which may lead to non-failure of students. This continues to be a matter of concern, as a major study exploring the reasons why mentors 'failed to fail' Nursing and Midwifery students in practice in the United Kingdom [Duffy 2004] and subsequent papers by Rutowski [2007] and Shapton [2007] show. Norcini [2005] concludes in his research with trainee general practitioners that it is not possible to make a fair assessment in a practice setting because the variables cannot be scientifically controlled. A constructive approach to assessment of practice is essential in order to produce healthcare professionals who are well prepared to step into the workplace [Clouder and Toms 2008]. Cowan, Norman and Coopamah [2005] conducted a literature review which concluded that a holistic approach is most conducive to assessing practice. The process should also contribute to the student's learning.

This study reports on the lived experiences of a group of students in their journey through practice learning and assessment towards qualification as practitioners in the fields of Social Work, Midwifery and Emergency Care (Nursing and Paramedicine). It took place over a four-year period, and was one of the strands of activity associated with the Centre for Excellence in Professional Placement Learning (Ceppl) at the University of Plymouth in the United Kingdom. An inter-professional research team of academics, practitioners, service-users and students from Social Work, Midwifery and Emergency Care informed the various stages of the study throughout its course. The diversity of the team enabled the members to reflect the understandings and perceptions of the various stakeholders, building on previous such experience [Elliot et al 2005].

A longitudinal case study approach was used to explore the students' experiences of practice assessment, with the focus of the research questions being on their perceptions of the validity and reliability of the methods used and the impact of the assessment process on their learning experience. A total of 14 students took part in semi-structured interviews which were held at the end of each academic year throughout their two to three year programmes. The longitudinal approach allowed the students' journeys to be seen in total rather than as a snapshot of an experience. This approach was also employed to enable the research team and student participants to build up a relationship throughout the study period, thereby optimising freedom of expression and richness of data.

For the purposes of this study, the research team developed generic definitions of the following key terms, drawing from a multi-professional workshop which preceded the main project:

- **Practice:** The application and development of the appropriate skills and knowledge to the professional role in the environment where that professional activity takes place.
- **Practice learning:** Distinguished by the framework of support, teaching and assessment for students on professional programmes, working alongside others to deliver a service to the public as part of their course.
- **Practice assessment:** May not necessarily take place in the clinical/ practice environment but must incorporate practice. Involves both formative and summative elements and includes all the evidence contributing to the judgement about whether the student can progress or not in practice.

Introduction

In order to clarify the different interpretations and various roles and practice assessment methods used in the three professional programmes, a glossary of terminology is provided in Table 1.

Table 1. Glossary of terms relating to assessment of practice

Term used	Professional group	Explanation
Assessor	Social Work	A qualified professional, who holds or is registered on the Practice Teaching Award who supports student learning and makes a judgement about the quality of the student's performance against the assessment criteria, including during the observations. An Independent Practice Assessor marks the summative portfolio.
CRAG (Criterion Referenced Assessment Grid)	Midwifery	A set of criteria against which the student is assessed. These comprise sets of key personal/ professional as well as clinical skills. The level to be achieved is based on Benner's "novice to expert", and gradually increases during the student's programme.
Mentor	Midwifery	A registered midwife with a mentorship qualification who facilitates the student's learning, supervises their practice and assesses them in the practice setting – completing documentation at identified points in the programme in the student's portfolio, particularly the CRAG.
Observation	Social Work	A pre-planned encounter with a service user/ carer (or group). The student prepares for this, is observed by an Assessor and receives feedback on the accuracy of their reflective self-assessment of their objectives and performance.
OSCE (Objective Structured Clinical Examination)	Emergency Care, Midwifery	A set of passive and/or active stations which are timed and assessed. These provide the student with a variety of opportunities for them to demonstrate to two assessors (usually one academic and one clinical) specific interpersonal and clinical skills.
Personal tutor	Midwifery, Social Work, Emergency Care	University lecturer who provides academic and pastoral support and monitors the student's clinical progress. In Midwifery this includes undertaking tripartite discussions at formative and summative points to 'moderate' the process of assessment
Portfolios	Social Work, Midwifery, Emergency Care	A compilation of evidence which comprises a range of materials depending on the programme being undertaken. These commonly include learning objectives/ outcomes, reflections, evidence of assessments (eg: observations in Social Work, clinical logs in Emergency Care, CRAG in Midwifery), progress reports or feedback from a variety of sources.

Table 1. (Continued).

Term used	Professional group	Explanation
Practice Learning Manager	Social Work	A qualified professional, who holds or is registered on the Practice Teaching Award who is the link between the student, agency and programme. Identifies learning needs and co-ordinates practice learning experiences to meet them. Responsible for overall management of the student's practice learning, but is not directly involved in assessment.
Practice Supervisor	Social Work	The individual in the placement setting who allocates work to the student and provides on-site day-to-day supervision and evidence to inform the assessment. Involved in the student's practice learning, but not directly involved in assessment.
Reflection	Social Work, Midwifery	A process of using knowledge to critically analyse practice experience, promoting learning from the situation and enabling the student to identify how it will influence their future practice.
Reflective log	Emergency Care	Structured reflections on practice demonstrating achievement of specific competencies.
Service-user/ carer	Social Work	Someone who has received a Social Work service themselves or for someone they care for. They participate in all aspects of the student's programme, from planning to initial conversations (prior to starting practice), to involvement in providing feedback, teaching and participation in assessment boards.
SLVT (Student Led Verification Tool)	Emergency Care	A practice-based assessment project. The assessment document comprises three themes. The student uses cues to guide the different aspect of the themes which more often than not is devoted to one subject. They can undertake a variety of subjects but the important aspect is that they are doing this theoretical or actual project in practice. Each theme is then written up and submitted for assessment.
Tripartite	Midwifery	A formal three-way discussion held between the student, their mentor and personal tutor. The purpose is to discuss progress at formative and summative points, provide guidance for future development and ensure that the criteria have been achieved.
Verifier	Emergency Care	A qualified health professional who guides and provides feedback to the student, and 'countersigns' their achievement of a practice action/s.

Chapter 2

METHODOLOGY

The aim of our study was to explore students' perceptions of the methods and processes used in the assessment of their practice throughout their professional programmes. The research questions were:

1. What are perceptions of validity and reliability of the practice assessment methods?
2. What are perceptions of the impact of the practice assessment process on the student learning experience?

Recognising that these views might well change over the two to three-year period of their programmes, a longitudinal case study approach was selected. Our rationale for choice of this qualitative approach was that it enabled complex phenomena to be explored from a range of perspectives, as the design allows for individual as well as multiple case studies to be examined. The advantage of a multiple as opposed to a single case approach is that evidence is considered more compelling and the study more robust [Yin 2003]. Case study design is predominantly used in the social sciences to provide an in-depth method of enquiry focusing on real life events. It is a methodology that is used across disciplines as diverse as Social Work and Management Science [Darke et al 1998]. Yin [2003] considers that case studies are valuable when considering the 'how' and 'why' questions of phenomena where the researcher has little control over events in given situations. The flexibility within the methodology enables real life practice to be explored and issues inherent in everyday practice to be addressed. It is therefore deemed to be particularly appropriate for practice based disciplines which are complex, in a state of constant flux and intrinsically linked to the social milieu of the discipline [Payne et al 2007]. Case studies are popular in educational projects to explore the experiences of individuals in educational settings in order to generate theory and move towards generalisation [Yin 2003]. Luck et al [2006] emphasise that it is the identification of the case/s to be studied that is crucial and that this must be decided and guided by the research question. In our research a case comprised firstly the individual student and their experience over the duration of their programme and secondly the student as part of the whole group of students.

In the case study approach, there is no statistical basis for sampling. The number of cases (or units of analysis) selected depends on the certainty the researcher wants [Yin 2003]. As the cohort numbers ranged from 15 – 90 students in the three professional programmes being studied, the research team decided to select five volunteer students from each. This enabled a range of placement areas to be represented, whilst ensuring the scale of the study remained manageable, as this approach is highly resource-intensive. It also allowed for some degree of attrition over the study period (ie: through withdrawal from the study, interruption or withdrawal from the programme) – whilst still protecting the multiple case element. A convenience sampling approach was taken [Frankfort-Nachmias and Nachmias 1996] – the invitation being extended to all students in the relevant cohorts during the first year of their programme. This took the form of an initial introductory email which was sent to all the students and was followed by a presentation visit by one of the research leads. A random number table was used to select five students from each cohort where more than the required number volunteered. There were no exclusion criteria. Ethical approval was obtained for the study.

The target groups were first year students on the following programmes at the University of Plymouth:

- Pre-registration Midwifery students undertaking the three-year BSc (Hons) Midwifery
- Pre-qualified Social Work students undertaking the three-year BSc (Hons) in Social Work
- Nurses and Paramedics undertaking the two-year post-registration BSc (Hons) in Emergency Care

Because of the nature of the Emergency Care programme (some students doing the full-time two-year degree whilst others undertook this in a part-time self-funded capacity extending over a period of up to five years) this was not a homogenous cohort. The participants were at varying stages of their programmes: two were coming towards the end of their part-time programme whilst the other two were in the first year of their full-time degree. Only four students were able to be recruited from this cohort. However, five students were recruited in their first year from both the Midwifery and Social Work programmes, resulting in a total of 14 participants.

The students were invited to take part in individual semi-structured interviews held at each annual summative assessment point, having first submitted their work. It was considered ethically important not to interfere with the assessment process itself, in order to avoid advantaging or disadvantaging the participants or other students. One of the students was referred in their final year, which meant that completion of the interviews was delayed until this student had also qualified. One student went on maternity leave in her third year which meant that we were unable to capture further data from this student, and another failed to attend for her final interview despite several appointments being made, with no explanation given. The interview data available from both of these students was, however, incorporated into the relevant year's findings. Table 2 shows the data relating to the number of interviews conducted with each participant. Of note, Emergency Care students were only recruited in the second year of the study due to their shorter programme, so only one or two interviews were conducted with this group.

The schedules for each set of semi-structured interviews were devised through consultation with the whole research team. In the first year these were based on the initial literature review and findings from a set of focus groups which had been held with final year students in the same three programmes prior to commencement of the longitudinal study. A report on this small exploratory study is in the process of being published [Fisher et al 2010]. In subsequent years the schedules were refined and developed, based on the emerging data from previous sets of interviews. The research team wanted to make best use of the longitudinal design, which enabled sequential interviews to be undertaken with the students and facilitated the identification of changed perceptions and development of the individual. Therefore in the final year some modification of the interview process was made. Not only were views on the current year wanted, but it was important to capture perceptions of the programme as a whole, in the context of practice assessment. Participants were sent the transcripts from their previous interviews as well as the final interview schedule in advance of the meeting. This enabled them to give deeper thought to the issues as well as helping them to compare their earlier and current perceptions. Several attended the interview with notes they had prepared, and commented favourably on this approach.

The interview team comprised the two lead researchers who were academics, two practitioners and one recently qualified student. Training of all members of the team was provided to ensure interviewer reliability [Silverman 1993, cited in Cohen et al 2000]. In an effort to reduce bias students were interviewed by a researcher who did not share the same professional background and/or was not previously known to the participant. The same student-interviewer partnerships were maintained throughout the duration of the study, which enabled a relationship of trust to be built up over the period and enhanced the depth of qualitative data obtained – a philosophy supported by Yin [2003].

Interviews were tape-recorded with the participants' written consent, and these were transcribed verbatim either by the interviewers themselves or research assistants employed by the Ceppl. Codes were used to protect anonymity. The transcripts were then emailed to the participants by their interviewer (ensuring confidentiality) in order to obtain member validation, and students were asked to add further comments as appropriate. They were also invited to request further informal interviews or contribute additional information via email at any point during the year prior to their next interview, should they wish to do so. During the four years of the study only one student requested an additional interview but several emails were received from other participants.

A general analytic strategy based on theoretical propositions was used in line with the case study approach. This involved pattern matching, explanation building and cross-case synthesis [Yin 2003, Miles & Huberman 1994]. The Framework technique devised by Ritchie and Spencer [1994] formed the baseline for single-case and cross-case analysis and synthesis of data. Thematic Content Analysis [Smith 1992] was undertaken independently by the two lead researchers after each round of interviews, and coding was cross-checked. Terminology used for themes and sub-themes was agreed through discussion. Findings were shared with the rest of the research team, and used to inform the subsequent interview schedules.

Table 2. Interview data (Shaded areas indicate interview undertaken this year)

Student code	Year one (2006)	Year two (2007)	Year three (2008)	Year four (2009)
ML1				Interviews completed
ML2			Referred – did not attend interview	
ML3				
ML4				
ML5				
S1			Maternity leave X2 years	
S2			Did not attend final interview	Interviews completed
S3				
S4				
S5				
EC1	Not recruited in the first round			
EC2				
EC3			No further interviews as programme completed	
EC4				

Chapter 3

FINDINGS

Three major themes emerged in the first round of interviews, and were strongly evident throughout the study. These comprised:

1. Process
2. Preparation
3. Purpose

Other themes were alluded to in the first year, and became more significant as the interviews progressed. There were some profession-specific differences in the timing and degree of importance of these issues to the participants. However by the final year they had become major themes to all professional groups. These were:

4. Placements
5. People
6. Professional persona

This chapter discusses the findings in the context of the stage in the students' programmes and their professional grouping. Discusssion is based on these six themes.

1. PROCESS

The methods used for practice assessment were explored at each interview. Questions were asked in relation to the students' perceptions of the reliability and validity of the various tools used. They were also probed on wider issues relating to the process of practice assessment. Some of the methods and tools were used in all professional groups and some were programme-specific. For ease of interpretation each is discussed individually in the context of the professional groups using the tool and changes to students' perceptions during their sequential interviews.

Portfolios

Portfolios were used in some format in all the programmes. Strengths included that they provided evidence of the student's capability and encouraged them as they could see their progress, giving them confidence. They also provided a focus and motivated their learning. One Midwifery student said how she

"loved the portfolio because it makes you think" (ML3).

Some students liked the self-directed components, although others were not sure that they were able to self-assess effectively. They were generally seen to be reliable and effective tools. Workload was a disadvantage – both the amount of time and forward-planning required to complete them and their physical bulk. One student suggested that electronic portfolios would be better. Emergency Care students were critical of the number of portfolios they were required to present.

Some Social Work students thought that their portfolios could be too prescriptive and weighting of marks was considered to be unbalanced. These negative aspects led to anxiety, and several students commented on elements which were viewed as *"ticking-box exercises"* which did not necessarily reflect their progress. The restricted expression through limited word-counts did not allow them to expand on and explore their learning. Several felt that they were unable to acknowledge some of their best work or the complexities entailed as there was nowhere to put this in their portfolio – just a *"list of work done"* (S3). This student went on to say that the need to *"jump through hoops"* and meet requirements meant that much of what was learned slipped away in the process of demonstrating the academic level required. One participant described it as

"parachuting bits of a jigsaw down a dark well" (S3)

and thought that it squandered the opportunity to recognise the student as a whole. There were also mixed views as to the appropriateness of having an unknown independent assessor marking their portfolios. Some saw this as consistent and objective, whereas others considered that these individuals lacked knowledge of the student and an appreciation of the context of their situation. Professional judgement of assessors was considered to vary. The portfolio caused a lot of anxiety to Social Work students and they wanted it to be more celebratory.

Some participants suggested that there was room for dishonesty in completion of their portfolios – there being the potential to *"cheat the system"* or *"blur the edges"*, thus making them unreliable – particularly highlighted in the Social Work and Emergency Care programmes. Potential for breaching confidentiality was also raised by both Midwifery and Social Work students. It was felt that the combination of first names of clients and some very unusual names for their babies could make them easily identifiable in the Midwifery portfolio.

However most students saw portfolios as a valid method of recording feedback from mentors and other staff with whom they worked. They appreciated comments being made which showed them where they could improve, and saw portfolios as a valuable method of demonstrating progress. They were generally viewed favourably and seen as a valuable reflective tool.

Reflections

Reflections were also used in all the programmes. These were generally deemed to be helpful, promoting growth and providing evidence of students' learning. All participants valued the process of reflection and felt that their skills in this area had developed, some having benefited from experimenting with a variety of structured models. One Social Work student commented that the increased opportunity to reflect in their second year portfolio had enabled them to demonstrate how their values had changed.

However reflections were generally seen as a very unreliable form of assessment. The sub-theme of 'twisting the truth' again emerged with frequency in both Social Work and Emergency Care programmes, and a Midwifery student stated that it was

"easy to write down what you think people want to hear" (ML3)

This view was demonstrated across all programmes and throughout the interviews. Concerns were also raised about issues of ethics and confidentiality. Some students said that reflections did not always evidence the reality of practice, and could be seen to be an exercise in *"ticking boxes"*. Emergency Care students stressed the importance of individuals choosing competencies which needed improving as topics to reflect on, rather than those which provided the line of least resistance. It was apparent that the effectiveness of reflections rested largely with the individual student's attitude and integrity.

OSCEs (Objective Structured Clinical Examinations)

Objective Structured Clinical Examinations (OSCEs) were used in both the Midwifery and Emergency Care programmes. This is a type of simulated practical examination used widely in medicine and other healthcare professions. All the students had found them to be very stressful and daunting, to the extent that some peers had been too nervous to attend on the day. The vast majority had, however, ultimately enjoyed them and felt they had benefited from this method of assessment. Most students thought that it was necessary to see how people behaved in a stressful exam situation. One Emergency Care student stated that he was wary of the argument that some peers felt unable to practise under clinical exam conditions, as they would have to be able to work and function in that type of environment. Students appreciated being able to demonstrate their knowledge and skills in a setting in which patients and clients were not being put at risk, particularly in emergency situations.

OSCEs seemed to particularly appeal to students who could liken the active stations to real-life practice (eg: Emergency Care Practitioners). However, some students considered that their typical practice was more holistic and that they did not verbalise their actions to the same extent in real life. It depended where the student's normal place of work was as to whether everyday practice was represented. One Emergency Care student thought that it was a very false environment which was alien and not holistic – saying that bits were missed out, and their ability to plan care was not picked up. Another likened it to *"playing a game"* (EC4). A Midwifery student expressed disappointment that they had not been tested in everything, considering that all high risk scenarios and emergencies should have been examined to ensure competence. She also suggested that it would be better to defer them to the third year when students had had more practice and were more confident. Some Emergency Care students were concerned if they were assessed by people they worked with, but Midwifery students liked the fact that their tutors could see them *"in practice"*. The OSCEs were rated highly for being consistent, fair, standardised, clear cut and professional and students liked their structured approach. Although some Emergency Care students had not been as enthusiastic in the first year of interviews, in the final round they clearly recognised the value of OSCEs as being able to inspire motivation and confidence and appreciated that this method tested safe practice. Participants considered that the tool engaged the students' learning and prepared them for emergency situations. It was identified as the one assessment which students really could not fabricate, and was therefore considered to be very reliable. Although stressful, the consensus was that it was an excellent tool which reflected practice and also formed a safety net for identifying incompetence.

Competence-Based Tools

Throughout their programme Midwifery students were continuously assessed through the use of the CRAG document (Criterion Referenced Assessment Grid) – a set of criteria statements identifying core clinical and professional skills which progressed along the lines of Benner's 'novice to expert' theory (1984). This tool was generally deemed to be reliable and provided guidance as to what needed to be assessed in practice. In the first year students found that the criteria were mostly achievable and focused their learning, however some were unrealistic and dependent on the placements the students were undertaking at the time. In subsequent years the weaknesses became more evident - particularly in relation to ambiguity and lack of clarity which could lead to variable interpretation of the *"woolly"* criteria, thus reducing their reliability. There was an element of subjectivity, and assessment depended on the honesty and professional judgement of the mentor. Some participants were aware of the changes which had already been made to the assessment tool in the new Midwifery curriculum – largely as a result of the concerns expressed during the longitudinal study – and were positive about the breakdown of the criteria into specifics, grading of practice and opportunity for comments guiding students on their progress.

In their first year the Midwifery students had also been required to complete a competence-based assessment tool which was commonly used throughout the Nursing programme in the institution. This comprised a set of performance criteria which had to be evidenced through at least two means. Students were very scathing of this in the initial round of interviews, criticising it for its unclear and unwieldy criteria and saying that they and their mentors had found it difficult, confusing, illogical and time-consuming to complete. However, interestingly, at the final interview a couple of the students said they would like more skills-specific assessments of this nature. Formal tests such as drug rounds would have also made the students feel more confident.

The Emergency Care programme used clinical logs as a competence-based assessment tool. These were on the whole viewed negatively, as they entailed a lot of paperwork and a large number of competencies. This was another form of assessment which seemed to be open to dishonesty as students said they could potentially make up these experiences because they were not always directly observed. One student described them as "*a bit dodgy*" (EC4). However, they did provide evidence of a range of skills.

Tripartites

Three-way meetings or tripartites were routinely undertaken in Midwifery and on occasions in both the Social Work and Emergency Care programmes. Although they could be difficult to arrange they were generally seen to be very helpful, providing a means of focusing learning and reflecting on progress. The meetings were perceived to be useful checkpoints and provided an opportunity for clarification of issues, constructive feedback and raising concerns. They were most reliable if the students had worked for a significant period of time with the mentor or communication had taken place with colleagues prior to the tripartite. Midwifery students found them to be generally transparent, supportive, relaxed and student-centred. However one participant likened the meetings to a "*parents evening*" or "*signing session*" (ML2). Some found it challenging to express conflicting opinions during the meeting, and it was suggested that the mentor and tutor should also have an opportunity for private discussion of the student's progress. One student remarked that comments during the tripartite had been at odds with previous feedback received from her mentor. Another said that she would have liked more *"feed-forward"* as comments such as *"this is fine"* were not particularly helpful. A third suggested that the process just gave a *"snapshot"* of a particular placement and mentor – both good and bad experiences of other placements could be missed out in the discussion. Tripartites were generally deemed to be helpful, and students valued the opportunity to hear out loud the thoughts of their mentor and personal tutor. It was suggested that an initial meeting with the mentor was also useful as it had helped to clarify learning objectives and expectations.

Although they were not a formal element of the Social Work programme, one student also commented on the value of *"three-way meetings"*, saying that these provided a good opportunity for feedback, created a balance between the student's self-assessment and others' interpretation, and that through these meetings they were able to turn incidents into learning experiences.

SLVT (Student-Led Verification Tool)

The Student-Led Verification Tool (SLVT) was a method specific to the Emergency Care programme. It comprised a structured practice-based project. All the participants initially found this tool daunting and difficult to understand, and would have valued being shown more examples and having a previous student reassure them that their anxiety was normal. However they learned a lot in the process and felt more prepared for its subsequent use. One student suggested that:

> "Maybe that's part of the educational process and maybe I needed to work out how to use it" (EC4).

This assessment method extended both academic and practice skills - but the degree of growth depended on the right subject being chosen which would be crucial to their practice. Students were pushed to research more widely and developed new strategies such as conducting a SWOT analysis or audit, whilst also

> "expanding their ability to work and write at degree level more than anything" (EC2).

Earlier use of this tool was suggested in order to develop these skills from the outset. Overall students enjoyed using the SLVT, which was thought to be structured and safe. During the course of the study some modifications were made to the tool, contributed to by our findings, and participants thought it had subsequently improved as explanations and the framework seemed clearer.

Observations

In their second and third years Social Work students had to undertake a specified number of direct observations. These were assessed by someone who did not normally work with them. Opinions varied widely regarding these. Some considered that observations were valuable, and they benefitted from the opportunity to prepare for them – although acknowledged that the time this took was unrealistic in the context of real-life work. Some students had to be creative in achieving their outcomes and set up situations which were not necessarily the norm. Some thought the observations reflected everyday practice such as interaction with the service-user and family, whereas others felt that they lacked authenticity due to the selection of a specific service-user to meet their needs and the amount of pre-planning involved. The process of being observed could also change the dynamics of the student-service-user interaction.

Some students struggled to organise appointments with their assessor or found it was not always a suitable time for the service-user. One student had experienced difficulties in prioritising whether to deal with a service-user need or complete their evaluation in their portfolio – a dilemma which had resulted in them putting the needs of the service-user first and reflecting in their portfolio why the evaluation was submitted late. On occasions service-users were in a situation where they were not *"voluntarily engaged"* (ie: prisoners) which could make conversation difficult. There was the suggestion that this was an area in which life or work experience could be beneficial in overcoming these issues. One student commented that their best work might not be observed as engagements with service-users could be too fragile, and considered that the fact that continuous assessment of practice didn't feature in the programme was a *"serious and significant failure"* (S3). It was suggested that a whole day of being shadowed while undertaking their normal activities would have been more authentic.

Observations were, however, deemed to be a more reliable form of assessment than portfolios and reflections as you couldn't *"twist the truth"* with them. They also gave the assessor a good insight into the student's practice and developed their learning. Students valued the feedback they received from a variety of sources, and the opportunity to reflect on the process with an experienced practitioner *"holding up a mirror to it"* (S3). Some students saw it as an advantage if they had more than one assessor for their observations as each could pick up on different issues and identify new learning needs, however others thought that this led to inconsistency. Inconsistency was also noted in guidance given and the level of experience of observation assessors. Placements, personalities of staff and their engagement with the role, as well as the student's own proactive approach contributed to the reliability and quality of the assessment.

Conversations

'Conversations' were held between the Social Work students and service-users as a means of ensuring their safety to practice in their first year. These were generally felt to be useful, providing a

> "thumbnail sketch of the student's person-centredness and communication skills" (S3).

Feedback was helpful. However, some students found this a *"nerve-racking experience"* and one considered that word limits for recording conversations *"short-changed the service-user"* (S1). They were also challenging to organise.

Presentations

Although the research team had not anticipated presentations being identified by the students as practice assessment tools through the preliminary work undertaken prior to the longitudinal study, several participants seemed to view these as such. One of the Midwifery students acknowledged their close links with practice. Emergency Care students had found their case study presentation to be highly pressured but beneficial, boosting their confidence and pushing them to the next level. Involvement in journal club presentations resulted in useful verbal and written feedback, and it was suggested that this could have formed part of the final mark. Students recognised that presentation skills were now more a part of their clinical work, such as patient handovers, as well as in their future roles as mentors.

General Comments on the Process of Assessment

Certain aspects of the assessment process were seen as 'facilitative', whilst others were 'obstructive'. 'Facilitative' aspects included:

- Assessors who had a clear understanding of the process and documentation and regularly supervised students.
- Direct observation of students' real-life practice, and not just a 'snapshot'.
- A general preference for grading to be undertaken to provide a benchmark, with a 'pass or fail' approach being less positively received. Students were keen that all elements of their practice should contribute to this grade, and that assessments should be marked individually to improve this benchmarking process.
- The overwhelming importance of constructive feedback was highlighted by all the participants throughout their interviews. This kept students on target, enabled clarification of expectations, confirmed skills and highlighted needs. It was very important to acknowledge the student's progress and help them to realise abilities they had not previously recognised. The timing of feedback was however vital, as if it was delayed the student could become demoralised or it would be too late to take into account suggestions made. Feedback comments also needed to match any mark given. Constructive feedback needed to be both verbal and written, and students wanted this to be detailed to enable them to develop. It was helpful if holistic reports came from a range of individuals including their mentor or assessor, personal tutor, other practice staff and the service-user. They acknowledged that some of the responsibility fell on themselves in being proactive and asking for specific feedback.

'Obstructive' elements to the process included inconsistent communication or mixed messages, lack of clarity about the correct way to use tools, unclear weighting of marks or expectation of milestones. Timing of portfolio submission could also be seen to be unfair or lacking in parity. Lack of time and workload were also factors which were 'obstructive' – some of the guidance given earlier was forgotten due to the sheer volume of the workload. At times there was a lack of clarity of the role of the assessor or their understanding of the assessment processes. Poor or delayed feedback, poor guidance by inexperienced supervisors, overpowering supervisors and inappropriate placing of students in situations where they felt out of control were seen to be unhelpful. Midwifery students had found the process wearing and stressful – particularly the constant scrutiny and time constraints.

When asked whether they thought that their practice which was being assessed reflected their normal practice, responses fell under four sub-themes:

- 'real-life',
- 'ivory tower',
- 'dark forest',
- 'jumping through hoops'.

Midwifery students were generally confident that their assessments reflected 'real life' and that their assessments were reliable. This was attributed by all students to the daily assessment, feedback and guidance they received through working closely with their mentors. One Midwifery student suggested that their true practice could only be assessed if they were shadowed all the time. Some Midwifery students barely recognised they were being assessed whilst others commented on the Hawthorn effect. One participant felt unsure about self assessment and another stated that the OSCE's might not reflect normal practice by being too controlled, thus coming under the heading of 'ivory tower' – although it was acknowledged that this was a necessary part of teaching *"correct skills"*.

In contrast, Social Work students were more ambivalent about their assessments reflecting normal practice. A few who drew from their past experiences considered that they were representative, some had their doubts ('dark forest') and others stated that there was too much of an emphasis on tasks and ticking boxes ('jumping through hoops'). The 'ivory tower' was a significant theme in this group. There were concerns about the normality and representative quality of the planned observations and some of the placements. The conversations with service-users in the first year of the Social Work programme were deemed to be artificial, and didn't reflect real practice. One student took the view that:

> "You're not assessed on your practice; you can practice superbly and you could fail the module, because what you're actually assessed on is

your perception to your practice, your recognition about how your practice has changed, and that is evidenced through the portfolio." (S3)

There was a real difficulty with being able to put complex situations into a restricted word-count. Some students said they tended to put on their best behaviour and exaggerated this to demonstrate that they were safe and respectful practitioners, however another said that they were able to overcome the Hawthorn effect. There was a general view that a longer period of observation would be preferable, with students being shadowed undertaking their daily work such as telephone conversations in order for real practice to be observed.

Emergency Care students thought that 99 percent of the time their 'real life' practice was being assessed, but that there was a risk that some students could make up procedures and cases for their clinical logs – there being a "*loophole for fudging*". Even though OSCEs were not typical practice as they were simulated, these provided valid evidence of the student's ability and safety. The students considered that assessment both influenced and reflected typical practice, thereby developing it. This student group differed from the other participants in that they were undertaking post-registration activity in their usual workplace, so were well aware of what 'real life' entailed.

Although participants across the programmes thought most assessment methods demonstrated achievement of learning, some required students to 'jump through hoops' and 'tick boxes'. In earlier interviews students had worried about these and the workload involved, but later on students valued the direction and focus they provided. This became accepted as part of the process by the final year, but they did need to have a clear purpose.

In the final interviews, participants were asked whether they thought that potentially unsafe practitioners could qualify with the practice assessment methods used in their programmes. Midwifery students were overall of the opinion that this was unlikely. The fact that they had worked with different mentors with different styles was seen as a safety-net. However, consistency of mentorship was key – if this was not available then it was more difficult for mentors to judge progress. Generally mentors seemed to be very aware of the accountability of their role – they wanted the students to do well but were concerned for the safety of their clients and very aware that the students were practising under their registration, so they were thorough in their supervision and assessment. Some participants had heard of peers who had been picked up as incompetent, and action was quickly taken – there being good communication between the mentors and the university tutors. However two had also heard of mentors who seemed prepared to sign anything, and the ambiguity of CRAG was also seen to be a risk factor. They were pleased that grading of practice was coming in, as they felt this would be an additional safety feature, and that mentors would make more considered opinions before signing students off.

Two of the Social Work students said there was definitely potential for unsafe practitioners to qualify, whereas a third thought that those people would get weeded out over the years. Risk factors were that there was nothing in the process which would find out if people were wilfully negligent, and the benchmark for passing was set too low. It was considered that people who were dangerous would not get through the assessment process, but borderline students certainly could. More of an emphasis needed to be placed on practical skills. Students highlighted the importance of triangulation of assessment in order to achieve reliability. There was a strong view that if just the portfolio was used as demonstration of practice competence this would cause concern.

Although Emergency Care students were generally happy with the assessment methods, they all had concerns about the potential for cheating. It was a very small risk, but present. They were dismayed that there were apparently plans to remove OSCEs from the programme, as they considered this tool to be a safety-net which would identify incompetence. It was known that plagiarism had occurred with assignments, and that clinical logs had been embellished – however one student concluded that this may not in fact always be a negative process as the student would still need to analyse the situation and anxieties, and consider how it would influence their practice in the future. It was unlikely that students could cheat in the SLVT as this was so complex and the tutors knew the subject so well that they could pick up on any problems. As in Social Work, the Emergency Care participants considered that triangulation of assessment methods increased reliability.

When asked what impact the practice assessment process had had on their learning, students generally responded that it had made a significant contribution. Students identified personal, professional and educational growth which was apparent from the first year and became even clearer by the end of their programmes. Most students talked about increased motivation, commitment and personal development. They considered that the assessment process reinforced existing experience and refocused learning. This resulted in them having an excitement at how the education process was moving them forward. The Midwifery and Emergency Care students clearly noted their progression and achieved a definite end-point. Social Work students had a less apparent structure. It seemed that they had reached a point on their journey rather than completion. All participants very clearly recognised the importance of life-long learning.

All the Midwifery students thought that the assessment process had enhanced their practice, although it had been an intense experience. Students had recognised their core skills and competencies and built on these, focusing around the CRAG criteria and addressing any gaps through proactive planning. This had become more structured as the years progressed and as the students moved towards an increased autonomy, taking responsibility and planning care. OSCEs were thought to have had a *"huge impact on learning"* (ML4), increasing their knowledge base and learning in practice. One student commented on their increased understanding of the point of reflection and the linking of practice and theory. They were unanimous in their view that the success of assessment lay in the experience and continuity of their mentor.

Social Work students were generally positive about how the assessment process had contributed to their learning, but there were also some criticisms. One participant identified negative aspects which included anxiety, concern and discomfort. Students felt that they had undertaken a steep learning curve in their first year and could see how far they had come both personally and professionally. They had developed reflexivity, the ability to question conflicts arising in practice and to determine their own levels of skill together with enhancing competence, knowledge and values. Students were more aware of self and other influences including politics, and had been pushed to do more research. Their confidence had increased and the relation between theory and practice had become clearer. One student had found it

> "empowering and liberating to bring in different knowledge to social work practice" (S3)

and he had been able to apply this to different areas of his work. One student felt they had learned more in their second than third year, and that their creativity had been stifled as the criteria had remained the same – seeing the third year as

> "a series of boxes to tick and hoops to jump through" (S4).

The observations had helped practice and improved participants' learning, but also slowed down their work. One criticised them as being *"snapshots"* which devalued the process of learning. It was suggested that if students could enjoy the observation process more rather than feeling they were *"ticking a box*" they would benefit more. One participant said they had lost sight of what they needed to learn as they were so busy concentrating on word counts, meeting requirements, presenting their portfolio to best advantage and selecting appropriate service-users for observations. They said it was not always possible to record in a portfolio what had been learned. Students were clear that the learning process is important – assessment should not be a *"tick-box"*. It was identified that if students were proactive they could develop their skills and take learning from most situations – but not all students in the group had been able to do this.

Emergency Care students had developed both practical and academic skills. OSCEs were a very clear favourite for developing their learning. The SLVT was likewise considered to have been very beneficial – new skills had been developed and the achievement of understanding had proved rewarding. Students felt motivated and enthused, and thought they could now contribute more to their work-place. There was a real sense of achievement. Assessment gave them direction and they realised the benefit of being motivated to improve their practice. They had valued formal feedback on their practice and found the development of their reflective skills very beneficial. They now self-assessed continually, questioning their practice and following up gaps in knowledge, enabling continuous professional development. They had found the experience of education liberating and were able to be more autonomous, confident and competent in their practice – *"It's a joy"* (FC2). One stated that it was *"like having been in a little box and allowed out"* (EC4). They thoroughly enjoyed sharing their knowledge with colleagues and felt empowered, which had in turn led to them being better able to empower peers and patients and promote good care. One of the students stated that assessment in the workplace was crucial to their role. They had learned to *"come from the right direction – safety first"* (EC4).

2. Preparation

Preparation and guidance were fundamental to the students' experiences across all professions and throughout the study. Their understanding of the 'process' and 'purpose' of practice assessment depended on sufficient preparation. All guidance needed to be seen to have a purpose and be relevant. Again, sub-themes of 'facilitative' and 'obstructive' guidance emerged.

'Obstructive' preparation and guidance was identified as inadequate clarity about expectations of the student or instructions regarding the various processes and methods used, incomplete information being provided in documentation, poor communication between the university and placement setting and inconsistency between verbal and documented guidance or information given by different people.

'Facilitative' guidance included provision of examples, detailed documentation, clear and consistent guidelines and face-to-face meetings such as pre-placement discussions with assessors and tripartite meetings during the placement.

In most cases materials were deemed to be clear and staff were supportive in clarifying issues. It was generally felt that information was given at the right time. Plenty of warning was given to students regarding the demands and stresses of the course. More written guidance was wanted on the expectations for reflections, portfolios, working agreements and clinical logs. However at times excessive guidance was provided which could be overwhelming and cause confusion and frustration. Some students stopped looking at the extensive information as despite being advised not to use it as a checklist they found this was unavoidable. Not all definitions and language were readily understood: "*Articulacy is actually a hindrance*" (S3), and this could cause confusion when trying to clarify a situation. Some staff supporting learners in the practice environment appeared to need more guidance about what was required of them or further explanation of assessment documentation. All outcomes needed to be very clear and explicit to avoid variations in interpretation or individual expectations and agendas.

There was an increased emphasis on the value of feed-forward in the final interviews. This included being shown examples of completed tools, sharing others' experiences and identifying areas for improvement. Some students suggested that earlier preparation pre-placement was needed, including its reality and complexities. One student commented that there had been poor communication between the university and the placement – the latter not expecting them and a supervisor not having been allocated. She suggested that a pack could have been sent to the area in advance. Where packs were used, such as in the Midwifery programme where one had been designed to assist them to make best use of non-maternity placements, this was identified as a positive experience, although not all the students had located or used this facility. Early in the programme, the students needed to be warned of the importance of keeping up with all assessments. They also thought it would be helpful to be able to speak to other students who had been through the process. Midwifery students would have appreciated regular guidance about the portfolio and detail of what was required, with specific criteria and milestones being highlighted each year. More information about what a tripartite comprised as well as expectations of the student-mentor relationship was wanted at the beginning of the programme. The value of pre-clinical and midpoint meetings with the mentor were highlighted, when interpretations of assessment criteria and expectations could be clarified. Workshops were provided on the observations, but some Social Work students found these lacked focus and were too late to be useful. It was also suggested that at least one observation should take place in the first year to "*demystify the process*". Emergency Care students commented that they would have benefited from more preparation for their OSCEs, and had valued student-initiated peer practice sessions and an explanatory DVD. They needed early access to practice OSCEs, and plenty of opportunities to rehearse them. They would have liked a formal mock examination. Students from all professions commented on the value of ongoing guidance. Not only was clear guidance and preparation needed prior to the placement, but regular rehearsal of the assessment methods and formative feedback was wanted, and was appreciated when it was received.

By the final year of interviews it was interesting to note how some students seemed to acknowledge that they couldn't actually have everything explained to them, and that they should not be spoon-fed. Some suggested that understanding how to undertake the assessments was perhaps a part of their learning - the very process of discovery seeming to contribute to the impact on their practice learning and personal development. One summed up the process of learning as:

> "If you don't go through the barrier, then you don't get the benefit of knowing what the benefit is" (EC4).

3. PURPOSE

Students were asked in each year what they thought was being assessed in their practice. Three sub-themes were evident throughout: Knowledge, Skills and Attitudes. The overlap between these and the existence of both inherent and learned factors resulted in two further sub-themes being identified:

a. Doing the job (knowledge and practical skills)
b. Being a professional (personal attributes and application).

There were some clear profession-specific differences in response to this question. In the first year the majority of comments related to 'doing the job' – particularly amongst the Midwifery students. Explanations for this may have been that several of the Social Work students had already had experience of working in a social care environment so would have already developed many of the core skills, or that this indicated the practical nature of Midwifery. It also reflected the different professional roles of the groups. Midwifery students predominantly referred to 'clinical skills', 'basic skills', 'evidence of ability' and 'active fulfilment of criteria'. The Social Work students, however, focused more on interpersonal skills such as 'negotiation', information handling', 'understanding' (of clients), 'interest' (in clients), 'empathy', 'conflict resolution' and the ability to determine situations. Both Social Work and Midwifery students identified similar aspects of 'doing the job' which included knowledge, application of theory to practice, ability and competence, rapport with clients, response to situations and team-working. All students highlighted the importance of listening, observation and communication skills.

In the second year the participants were specifically asked what they considered to be the point of practice assessment. It was evident in this round of interviews that the students had a clearer recognition of the purpose of practice learning and its assessment. They had moved on from 'doing the job' to 'being a professional', suggesting that not only was their ability to do the job being assessed but also their suitability for the profession. There was a clearer understanding of the links between theory and practice, and students were able to apply their knowledge more effectively. 'Self-awareness' and 'reflective ability' were recognised as being important attributes as well as confidence to undertake the role.

Midwifery students were particularly conscious of needing to learn the skills which were required to become a safe, knowledgeable, professional and competent practitioner, with the necessary clinical abilities. They were building on existing skills and acquiring new ones as well as applying transferable skills to other settings. They were linking theory with practice and thinking holistically. They considered that practice assessment tested this knowledge and ability as well as providing guidance on how their practice should be developed. Students stated that they were being assessed on their midwifery practice and ability to cope with real life situations. They realised that this not only provided them with the opportunity to achieve the programme requirements but also enabled them to work towards a professional qualification. It appeared that the knowledge learned to 'do' the job, in both groups then fed into the ability to apply this knowledge to 'being' professional.

Social Work students were likewise very conscious of the importance of safety and competence as a practitioner, and considered that the assessment judged their ability to practice within a "*safety net*". There was an emphasis on self-awareness - critical analysis of their own practice, recognising limitations and how to address these, the way they approached life and personal attributes. Assessment of interactions with service-users was important, as evidenced in the observations. Students recognised that they needed to gather their skills such as communication and increase their knowledge, integrating these into practice. They thought their practice learning developed their ability to use skills and language without consciously thinking about them. They were being assessed on their ability to monitor risks as well as their own values such as their approach towards issues of authority/ gender/ class/ race. They valued the objective feedback they received as a means of improving their practice. They considered that assessments tested ethical practice and their ability to put theory into practice, developing the 'art' of becoming a social worker.

Emergency Care students were only interviewed for the first time in the second year, but because they were already registered healthcare professionals, their responses were more similar to the later interviews with the Midwifery and Social Work students. They outlined a range of personal and professional skills which were developed during their programme. These included autonomy, clinical leadership, critical analysis of actions, assessing and planning skills, communication skills and the ability to relate to the client, reassure them and take histories, clinical governance, depth of understanding, approach, performance and ability to undertake clinical skills. Safety and competence were identified as well as self-awareness – "ability to know ability" and gaps in knowledge. One student commented that the complete health care professional was being assessed, with the bigger picture being viewed. The students commented favourably on their University programme compared to the "*number-crunching method of assessment in the ambulance service*" (EC2) which was an ongoing check on competence. Students considered that their Emergency Care programme brought a different perspective to the assessment of practice, with there being more of an emphasis on what was learned than what was taught.

In the final round of interviews all the students were very clear on what was being assessed, and were very aware of the professional end-point. Most stated competent clinical and professional performance which demonstrated that they were ready for qualification and registration. The ability to practise autonomously and safely, demonstrating the ability to make decisions, problem solve and cope with stress was mentioned by all professional groups. The application of knowledge and professional values to real practice was also highlighted. All students clearly *wanted* to be assessed in practice

In the final year, when asked who they thought they needed to please in order to achieve in their practice assessment, nearly all students identified the assessor, self, the service-user and academic staff. Students rationalised and gave differing priority to these. Mentors and practice assessors needed to ensure the student was safe and met the criteria. Academics needed to ascertain that the student was following due process – two Social Work students said they needed to tick the university boxes. Across the range of professions, some participants identified that the service-user was the first person to make happy and this was more important than the student's practice assessment experience. In fact one Social Work student went so far as to say that they were not trying to please anyone, but were trying to find the right outcome for the service-user. Students wanted to please themselves by performing well and meeting their own expectations – it was important to prove that they were safe, competent practitioners.

The differences between the groups' identification of knowledge and skills may well support the argument that even though there may be generic principles of assessment, a profession-specific component is likely to be needed in order to meet the requirements of each professional role.

4. PLACEMENTS

Placements were seen as a major factor in Social Work and Midwifery student programmes. These could greatly affect practice learning and assessment experiences. Appropriateness of the placement setting and timing in relation to practice assessment was very important. Variations between placement experiences and levels of support in these could impact on the student's learning as well as their ability to achieve the required elements of the assessment. The nature of the service where the students practised also had an impact on their ability to conform to the assessment processes. In both professions inconsistency of placements meant students had differing experiences, which affected their learning. There were also concerns about availability of sufficient placements.

Not all placements contributed to the students' understanding of what Social Work really entailed. Some were useful but others lacked clear purpose, were inappropriate and disorganised and caused conflict. In one the milestones had changed during their placement which also had health and safety implications for the student. Some Social Work students had found it difficult to link the practice learning module outcomes with their placements and not all had met their learning or assessment needs. Although issues around placements (such as whether they were in the statutory or voluntary sector) could impact on experience and learning, one student said they had learned to deal with the challenges and complexities of their placement, using setbacks as a positive experience.

Timing of placements in relation to summative points and their location had a significant influence on the Midwifery students' experiences, there being a wide geographic spread of placements. The ability of assessments to reflect typical practice depended on a student's placement at the time. The CRAG statements were not always attainable in every placement, and students sometimes needed to access alternative clinical areas to achieve the criteria. When students worked on labour ward this gave a correct impression of how they were in practice because they worked with a midwife all the time, whereas on the postnatal or antenatal ward more autonomous working meant that they were not always observed in their work and interaction with women. Consistency of mentoring was found to be more difficult to achieve in the hospital than the community setting. Likewise, it was more difficult for students to be directly observed in hospital due to staff shortages. A placement in a gynaecology ward was deemed *"fantastic"* (ML5) as this had been *"wonderful in rounding out nursing skills"* as well as providing the opportunity to work in a different team environment. One Midwifery student thought that it was an advantage to work in a single clinical area as her capabilities were then better known and she was given more opportunities to undertake wider learning experiences.

Placement issues did not appear to be such a concern for Emergency Care students. This was probably because most were already employed in the relevant areas – although one did comment that she had to seek specific experiences elsewhere in order to meet the programme needs.

5. PEOPLE

The person supporting the student in practice was seen as crucial in all three professions. They were the gatekeeper enabling the student to gain the experiences they needed and achieve the required elements. The student's relationship with this individual was crucial.

The attributes of the assessor in all programmes were also significant. These centred around their professionalism, accountability, personality and experience. One Midwifery student stated that a good mentor could not be fooled. Their values and beliefs, professional judgement and accountability were vital. Their knowledge and ability to undertake a reliable and fair assessment and give constructive feedback were essential to enable the student to develop and meet the required competencies. In one case a Social Work student commented on receiving poor feedback and commitment from their Practice Learning Manager which made them anticipate failure. Their attitude to the role was very important – a disinterested, inexperienced or over-controlling assessor could create a very negative experience for the student. Inconsistency between their approaches, styles or perceptions of requirements could also cause problems. Staff needed to take their role seriously and engage effectively with the student as well as liaise with practice and academic colleagues regarding their progress. They also needed to be aware of other conflicting demands on the student such as the interplay between practice and academic burdens. Students wanted them to be supportive and good listeners. Mentors and assessors needed to be well prepared for their roles.

Midwifery students thought that consistency of working with their mentors was vital. Continuity with the main assessor allowed them to note the student's progress, know their capabilities and build up trust, enabling them to "*back off*" so that their normal practice could come through. However if the mentor and student did not know each other well, this could result in the student being over-supervised in their third year when they wanted to demonstrate that they could "*fly*". It was also important that the mentor knew the student well as they might otherwise assume that they were at the same level as other students in the year whereas in fact they may be struggling. One student commented that the advantage of having fewer mentors was that she did not have to keep starting again when working with someone new, and there were increased opportunities for their mentor to see them working in similar circumstances on more than one occasion. Emergency Care students also considered that there was real value in the continuity of the clinical assessor as they could more easily identify improvement. Social Work students verbalised that they would prefer more frequent, regular and extended contact and observation which reflected everyday practice rather than having artificially set up assessments. They expressed a desire for consistency in their Practice Learning Supervisor.

In contrast most students also identified the importance of others being involved in their assessments. They appeared to desire a triangulation of views as this could improve practice, increase reliability and provide a safety-net for detection of poor practice. A range of professionals in both practice and academic settings already contributed to the assessment of students. In addition, service-user feedback was part of the Social Work programme. All students welcomed contributions from others, stating that this created a balance - however one Social Work student commented that more than enough people were already involved in assessing their practice, but the way in which this occurred needed to change. Both Midwifery and Emergency Care students wanted contributions from a wider range of professionals such as consultants and staff from other health professions. Emergency Care participants were particularly keen on a more structured model of mentorship for reflection and advice. It was noted by Midwifery students that if they had worked with more than one mentor it would be helpful to have them contribute formally or attend the tripartite to give a more realistic view of the student, as one student said that information about other experiences wasn't always being relayed. Some of the participants also expressed a wish for greater contact with other students. This could include sharing of experiences of assessment methods and tools, demonstration that they had "survived" the process, teaching junior students, group discussions and mutual feedback. Although most students were keen on the involvement of service-users or clients and perhaps peers in their practice assessment, this did also raise concerns regarding a potential conflict of interests. Students were generally positive about the support they received from their academic tutors. Academic input to practice was explicit in Midwifery and Emergency Care, but only seemed to take place if there was a problem in Social Work – however a positive relationship with the Practice Learning Manager could enhance these students' experiences. Effective communication between university and placement staff was seen as vital.

6. PROFESSIONAL PERSONA

This theme began to emerge in the first round of interviews but became much more significant as the students progressed through their programmes. In the first year Midwifery students were aware of political professional issues, some of which impacted on them personally whilst there was also recognition of the wider role of the midwife. Shortage of staff and budgetary cuts affected some students' practice experience, resulting in a feeling that they were being "*used*". There were also concerns about role changes resulting in skill loss for qualified midwives (eg: the Midwifery Support Worker taking away their holistic role).

In the second year all participants were developing a 'professional persona'. Midwifery students emphasised the importance of developing confidence and competence, enabling them to become safe and autonomous practitioners. They thought that the consolidation of practice prepared them for work in the real world, and expressed the hope that they would be given even more responsibility the following year. They were conscious of the level of accountability in what could be a very high risk environment. They were also mindful of the responsibility of and onus on being a mentor. Overall, the perceptions of Midwifery students with relation to practice assessment seemed to have changed - either through personal circumstances, professional development or their experience of the assessment process. This led to greater awareness of the importance of acquiring practice competence versus theory success. Midwifery students were keen to have weaknesses identified and not to be automatically passed in practice. They acknowledged that "*learning is phenomenal in two years*" (ML3) and that it was very hard work, but it had all "*clicked this year*" (ML3). The people they worked with seemed to have more faith in the students' abilities, and all experiences had added to their confidence.

Many Social Work students had become more skilled at reflecting on their practice. One said she wanted to

> "develop into a particular type of practitioner with individualistic style who is able to go above and beyond the social work literature to create an appropriate form of practice which transcends the way social work is moving at the moment" (S4)

and another thought that their practice learning should develop an "*insightful practitioner*" (S5).

Although it was the first year that Emergency Care students were interviewed, their range of experience varied and some were already at the end of their programme. This, together with the fact that they were already qualified practitioners undertaking post-registration studies, seemed to result in them having a much clearer understanding of the need for a professional approach. They knew their limitations and saw this as a strength, valuing the opportunity to practise and develop in identified weak areas. One student said their learning had *"hugely enhanced [my] ability to go out and give people the right care pathway they need"* (EC3).

There was clear development of the professional persona in the final interviews. Students were much less focused on themselves and more aware of their peers and the wider context in which they were practising. They were clearly able to verbalise aspects which needed improvement. The individual's values and personality were recognised as impacting on the professional they would become. There was a marked difference between the students who had had previous experience in the professional roles and those who didn't. Both the Emergency Care students and the Social Work students who had previously had experience considered that the programme and assessment processes had enhanced their skills and values as well as teaching them new ones. The Midwifery students, however, seemed to demonstrate a much more structured and progressive development of their skills during the programme. All the students took responsibility for their own development and achievement. Poor experiences of placements or individuals were used positively and blame was not laid.

In the final interviews students were specifically asked in what ways the practice assessment had contributed to them becoming a professional, ready to qualify. Midwifery students were positive about the contribution the practice assessment process had made. They identified focus and consolidation of learning, huge personal development, gaining confidence, being made to think and being able to shine in one area if they did not have skills in another. The process gave them structure in their placement and the things they needed to learn. They said that it was crucial that they had as much practice as they did, and that this ran throughout the course. One had benefited from seeing a lot of integrated team practice, and they had got to know people and learned to function in a multidisciplinary team. They had been able to notice the difference in themselves – although it seemed a slow process they looked back and realised how far they had come. They had tried to become more specific in ensuring they met their landmarks, picking up on gaps. Progress statements in their portfolio were good to read through. They had found feedback from everyone – academics, mentors, other staff, women they cared for – very constructive, and said that this had mostly been tactfully given. One Midwifery student identified the importance of knowing her limitations and feeling ready before being signed up as competent.

Emergency Care students had found their knowledge and confidence hugely boosted. It had made them a more professional practitioner by enhancing existing practice, smoothing off the edges and making them more well-rounded and dynamic. Evidence-based practice techniques were demonstrated through their practice, and they were constantly updating themselves – the assessment process had encouraged them to research and think for themselves. They wanted to improve continually, and were more autonomous practitioners.

Similarly, some of the experienced Social Work students thought that it had guided and refined their practice, defined their values, provided them with an academic base and enabled them to be agents of social change. It had become clear what they wanted to be, and did not want to be. Challenging experiences had taught students not to respond in a knee jerk fashion or take things personally. Students had become more reflective and self-critical.

Of interest, one student in each of the three professional groups had advanced further in that they were considering their future role as a mentor – either having already committed themselves to becoming one or putting themselves in their assessor's shoes and considering how they might supervise students in the future.

The loopholes for validity and potential to "*twist the truth*" continued to be concerning. Although it is recognised that students will inevitably choose the easy option at times, it is still worrying that these are potential (or existing) professionals and it raises questions about accountability. However the reassuring aspect was that the participants clearly disapproved of such practice, and felt there should be tighter measures to prevent this. They wanted the borderline students to be detected and addressed, and were pleased when this took place.

Other Findings

In the final round of interviews, participants were asked whether they thought that it was appropriate or indeed possible to measure aspects such as confidence, motivation, attitudes and professional identity. This question gained mixed responses from all professional groups. Many students felt that these aspects were inherent in the student's personality and assessment of them as individuals. Some thought this was already sub-consciously undertaken through the overall assessment, and was enhanced by continuity of an assessor who could note improvements. Although some aspects were easier to identify such as motivation and a positive attitude it was more difficult to measure confidence. Not all students were equally confident but could be equally competent. Generally students didn't think that professional identity could be measured, although there was some potential for this in the reflective portfolios, and a Social Work student thought that this developed in the third year. Most students thought these aspects could not be summatively measured, but could be a part of formative assessment – however this should not be in a critical manner. It was generally thought than any measurement would be likely to be subjective, and could not be broken down into a set of statements or tick-boxes. One Emergency Care student thought a non-invasive measurement such as a scale of nought to five could be helpful – with it being contributed to by the assessors and themselves. It would, however, be a very changeable measurement and it would be difficult and probably not helpful to mark. Another suggested that motivation and attitude should be criteria for selection for the course. A Social Work student said that psychometric testing should be undertaken for all potential students. It was also suggested that tutorials, student presentations, group activities, demonstration of professional behaviour and competent practice in the work-place and reflective portfolios already assessed these aspects.

A number of issues contributed to conflict for the students in all programmes. There were concerns about availability of sufficient mentors and placements in more than one programme. Some Social Work students had experienced dilemmas associated with the needs of the service-user versus their own. There had been a power struggle between one of the participants and her assessor. Some Midwifery students found the level of intense scrutiny they had experienced by being continuously assessed by their mentor wearing:

> "It has been the most intensive, extended period of intrusive scrutiny of my entire life – it's like being assessed everyday... and it's so, they're so testing your personality as well as your clinical practice that you just feel pulled apart the whole time... I do think mentors need to appreciate it's a really tough course. It's very, very full time and it's exhausting" (ML1).

Several Social Work students commented on how hard the course had been, and how it had *"taken over your whole life"* (S2). Many of the participants had been challenged by the juggling of time between personal life and the course, and academic and practice demands. Both Midwifery and Emergency Care students had experienced difficulties with the attitude of clinical staff who were not always empathetic about the fact that the student was both doing clinical shifts and studying towards a degree. This was particularly the case in Emergency Care where the relatively new programme had been viewed with some suspicion by colleagues who had challenged the students, initially finding it difficult to understand why they were doing the course – though by the final interviews some had expressed an interest in undertaking it themselves! However students were generally positive about the level of support they had received, and were very pleased that they had achieved.

Chapter 4

CONTEXTUALISING OUR RESEARCH STUDY

Having followed the chosen methodology of a longitudinal, multi-professional case-study approach, we were keen to ascertain how this had contributed to the body of evidence in the context of assessment of practice. A comprehensive review of the most recent literature published in the English language during the course of our study from 2006 until the start of 2009 was therefore undertaken in order to view the trends in the most current research, evaluation and debate within the area of practice assessment. Relevant databases were searched in order to ensure diverse coverage of international literature in terms of professional focus, research and evaluation methods and practice assessment definitions relating to health education, Social Work, Nursing, Midwifery and field education.

Thirty-nine papers in this period specifically or broadly evaluated the assessment of practice and/ or practice assessment tools. The papers were reviewed in order to determine firstly the professional focus, secondly the extent to which tools used for assessing practice were evaluated by the literature and thirdly the methodology used. A summary of papers can be found below, in Table 3.

Table 3. Summary of current evidence

Category	No. of papers	References	Comments
PROFESSIONAL FOCUS			
Uni-professional	34	Brosnan et al. (2006) Byrne & Smyth (2008) Cassidy (2008) Dearnley & Meddings (2007) Ghaye (2007) Hobden (2007) Kear & Bear (2007) Kevin (2006) Kneafsey (2007) Kneafsey & Haigh (2007) Lauder (2008) McCarthy & Murphy (2008) McCready (2007) McMullan (2006) McMullan (2008) Nairn et al. (2006) Pirie & Gray (2007) Rushforth (2007) Rushworth (2008) Speers (2008)	Nursing (n=20)
		Crisp et al. (2006) Clare (2007) Hay & O'Donoghue (2008) Humphrey (2007) Swigonski et al. (2006)	Social Work (n=5)
		Davis et al. (2009) Lewis et al. (2008) Vnuk et al. (2006)	Medicine (n=3)
		Clouder & Toms (2008) Coote et al. (2007) Hadfield et al. (2007)	Physiotherapy (n=3)
		Jay (2007)	Midwifery (n=1)
		Abbey (2008)	Osteopathy (n=1)
		Sharpless & Barber (2009)	Clinical Psychology (n=1)

Category	No. of papers	References	Comments
Multi-professional	4	Atwal et al. (2008)	nursing; health care assistants; occupational therapists; physiotherapists
		Clemow (2007)	post-registration nursing; paramedics; physiotherapists
		Dunworth (2007)	social work; post qualified nursing
		London (2008)	osteopathy & medicine
Generic	1	Johnson (2008)	
ASSESSMENT TOOLS EVALUATED			
Portfolios	11	Atwal et al. (2008) Davis et al. (2009) Ghaye (2007) Hadfield et al. (2007) Kear & Bear (2007) Lewis et al. (2008) McCReady (2007) McMullan (2006) McMullan (2008) Nairn et al. (2006) Swigonski et al. (2006)	
OSCEs	4 (+1)	Brosnan et al. (2006) Byrne & Smyth (2008) Jay (2007) Rushforth (2007)	
OSCEs (cont)		Lauder (2008)	Did not evaluate efficacy of tool per se; employed the tool to measure competence
Other tools	3	Abbey (2008)	Final Clinical Competence Assessments and Clinical Tutor Reports

Table 3. (Continued).

Category	No. of papers	References	Comments
		Pirie & Gray (2007)	Competency assessment tool aimed at assessing the administration of blood components.
		Coote et al (2007)	Common assessment form for physiotherapy students
METHODOLOGICAL APPROACH			
Qualitative	11	Byrne & Smyth (2008) Clare (2007) Clemow (2007) Clouder & Toms (2008) Dunworth (2007) Hay & O'Donoghue (2009) Humphrey (2007) Jay (2007) Kneafsey (2007) McMullan (2008) Speers (2008)	Focus groups, Interviews, Document analysis, Questionnaires (open-response)
Quantitative	9	Abbey (2008) Coote et al. (2007) Kear & Bear (2007) Kneafsey & Haigh (2007) Lauder et al. (2008) Lewis et al. (2008) McMullan et al. (2006) Nairn et al (2006) Vnuck et al. (2006)	Scales, Questionnaires, Analysis of student grades, Tool development
Mixed methods	6	Brosnan et al (2006)	focus groups & questionnaires
		Pirie & Gray (2007)	surveys & interviews
		Davis et al. (2009); McCarthy & Murphy (2008)	questionnaires with open and closed questions

Category	No. of papers	References	Comments
		Dearnley & Meddings (2007)	included analysis of researcher memos
		Atwal et al. (2008)	structured observations
Literature review	4	Crisp et al. (2006) Hadfield et al (2007) McCready (2007) Rushforth (2007)	
Position/discussion paper/commentary/editorial	8	Cassidy (2008) Ghaye (2007) Hobden (2007) Johnson (2008) Kevin (2006) London (2008) Sharpless & Barber (2009) Swigonski et al. (2006)	
Reflections on study tour	1	Rushworth (2008)	

- **Professional focus** – In comparison with our study which had involved Midwifery, Social Work and post-registration Nursing and Paramedic students, all but three of the 39 papers reviewed were uni-professional in focus, with by far the greatest number of papers (20) solely targeting the assessment of Nursing practice.

- **Assessment tools evaluated** - Portfolios (reflective, electronic and paper-based) were the most widely evaluated tool, which reflected our study in which all three programmes had used this method. Four of the reviewed papers evaluated OSCEs and three other tools used to assess practice including Final Clinical Competence Assessments and Clinical Tutor Reports. Remaining papers focused on what can be described as key areas or issues relevant to the assessment of practice, such as the involvement of others in student assessment, grading and the assessment of specific competencies.

- **Methodological approach used** – Only 11 of the 26 original research papers utilised purely qualitative methods in the form of interviews and focus groups, thematic analysis of learning outcomes documentation and open-response questionnaire items. Six studies used mixed methods such as questionnaires and focus groups, while the remainder used purely quantitative methods.

Our choice of qualitative methodology using a longitudinal case-study approach and involving a range of health and social work programmes was therefore unique, producing rich and varied data which has significantly contributed to the current body of evidence in the context of assessment of practice. It enabled an extended view to be taken of the student experience, which has provided a richness of data which a 'snapshot approach' would not have achieved. A level of trust was built up between the interviewers and participants which enabled the latter to demonstrate a surprising level of openness about some of the issues raised.

The longitudinal approach has enabled single-case as well as cross-case analysis to be undertaken. Diverse representation in the study group has provided valuable insights into the strengths and weaknesses of a range of assessment tools and methods across a variety of professions. It is hoped that some of the findings and recommendations of this research will be of benefit to a number of professional programmes.

Many of the students commented on the value of having been part of the study. This had not only benefitted them, but also their peers who had used the interviews as a conduit of communication with the programme teams. Several students had appreciated the opportunity to debrief and "*off-load*" at the end of each year with a trusted third party. They had been appreciative of the programme changes which had already been made – some as a direct result of the feedback received during the interviews. They had been enthused by their involvement in the decisions which were made and had enjoyed being a part of the research.

The final round of interviews provided a wonderful opportunity not only to review the last year of the students' programmes, but to gain an overview of their individual journeys which had got them to the point of qualification and professional registration. A greater balance of opinions was apparent as the students had progressed beyond the initial stages to a new place of understanding and professionalism.

Chapter 5

RECOMMENDATIONS

Although this study had its limitations – for example incomplete data sets and variable interviewing experience within the team – the longitudinal design seemed to overcome these to an extent. A particular strength was that findings did not rely on a 'snapshot' of experience, and changed perceptions were able to emerge in subsequent interviews. Some students indicated that they had consulted peers on their views and incorporated these into the discussion. This increased generalisability of the findings. Although it is acknowledged that these only reflect student views which may on occasions differ from staff opinions, the purpose of practice learning and assessment should not be overlooked. If students believe that these suggestions would contribute to their learning and optimise reliability of assessment, then consideration should be given to embedding them into professional programmes.

Some very specific assessment tools were used in the programmes studied, however key principles emerged which may be translated to a range of methods and professional groups. A set of generic recommendations has therefore been developed based on our findings and the suggestions from students, which may be seen below (Table 4).

What more heartening conclusion to a programme can there be than when a student says, in the words of one of our Emergency Care participants (EC2):

> "A colleague of mine summed it up nicely when we started. He said the thing about the degree isn't really arriving at the end with a tick in the box, it's the journey that's the most important thing and you do get out of it what you put in.... That journey, it was great as far as I was concerned"

Table 4. Recommendations for practice assessment

Preparation and feed-forward	<ul><li>Early and ongoing guidance</li><li>Timely guidance</li><li>Prepare students for placement to optimise experience</li><li>Students know placement in advance</li><li>Placement expects student and receives information pack</li><li>Vetting of placement and assessors</li><li>Opportunity for students to practise skills in a controlled setting</li><li>Opportunity to rehearse assessment methods</li></ul>
Flexibility	<ul><li>Avoid 'ticking boxes'/ prescriptive elements without a clear purpose</li><li>Scope for individuality in assessment</li></ul>
	<ul><li>Word counts need to enable students to expand on and explore learning</li><li>Flexibility in submission dates</li><li>Choice in placement</li><li>Alternative assessments (eg: discussion/ viva, accredited learning, electronic portfolio, direct observation, peer assessment)</li></ul>
Clarity	<ul><li>Explicit, written guidance</li><li>Specific criteria</li><li>Examples</li><li>Talk to previous students</li><li>Clear moderation process</li><li>Clarity of expectations (eg: relationship with assessor/ milestones)</li></ul>
Consistency and reliability	<ul><li>Assessment directly relevant to placement context</li><li>Parity of experience across cohorts/ placement contexts</li><li>Assessment throughout placement – avoid snapshots</li><li>Consistency and continuity of support and assessment throughout programmes/ placements</li><li>Use all available evidence</li><li>Triangulation of assessment methods/ people</li><li>Final marker should input into assessment throughout year/ placement</li><li>Uniform training processes for assessors</li><li>Experienced assessors</li></ul>
Contact and communication	<ul><li>Increased contact between university and placement staff</li><li>Written contract between university and placement</li><li>Increased placement visits by academics</li><li>Action learning sets for students in placement to share experiences</li></ul>

Involvement of others	• Triangulation of views • Increased involvement of others to enhance reliability and authenticate assessment (eg: service-users/ clients, peers, academics, managers, other placement staff) • Opportunity to shadow others
Feedback	• Frequent meetings with clinical assessor • Formative checkpoints/ three-way meetings for feedback • Consistency in assessor/ person providing feedback • Consistency between feedback and grade awarded • Comprehensive record-keeping regarding progress • Specific, written feedback • Good, unbiased, reflective, before and after events/ placement, regular • Assessor to feedback on specific and broader issues • Students to proactively seek specific feedback • Guidance on how to improve • From a range of individuals for balance
Formalised assessment	• Direct observation • Increased formal clinical assessment to ensure competence • Self-assessment and assessment by others • Grading of practice • Balance between practical and academic assessments • The learning process is important

ACKNOWLEDGMENTS

Avril Bellinger, Mark Berry, Anne Binns, Susan Eick, Janet Leeds, Julie Mann, Miriam McMullan, Lauren Mutton, Yvonne Strutt, Marie Turner, Daniel Webster, Emma Whittlesea and the student participants

REFERENCES

Abbey, H. (2008). Assessing clinical competence in osteopathic education: analysis of outcomes of different assessment strategies at the British School of Osteopathy. *International Journal of Osteopathic Medicine*, *11*, 125-131.

Atwal, A., Tattersall, Caldwell, K., Craik, C., McIntyre, A. & Murphy, S. (2008). The positive impact of portfolios on health care assistants' clinical practice. *Journal of Evaluation in Clinical Practice, 14*, 172-174.

Benner, P. (1984). *From novice to expert: Excellence and power in clinical nursing practice.* Menlo Park: Addison-Wesley.

Brosnan, M., Evans, W., Brosnan, E. & Brown, G. (2006). Implementing objective structured clinical skills evaluation (OSCE) in nurse registration programmes in a centre in Ireland: A utilisation focused evaluation. *Nurse Education Today, 26*, 115-122.

Byrne, E. & Smyth, S. (2008). Lecturers' experiences and perspectives of using an objective structured clinical examination. *Nurse Education in Practice, 8,* 283-289.

Cassidy, S. (2008). Subjectivity and the valid assessment of pre-registration nurse clinical learning outcomes: Implications for mentors. *Nurse Education Today, 29(1),* 33-39.

Chambers, M. A. (1998). Some issues in the assessment of clinical practice: a review of the literature. *Journal of Clinical Nursing, 7(3),* 201-208.

Clare, B. (2007). Promoting deep learning: A teaching, learning and assessment endeavour. *Social Work Education, 25(5),* 433-446.

Clemow, R. (2007). An illuminative evaluation of skills rehearsal in a mentorship course. *Nurse Education Today, 27,* 80-87.

Clouder, L. & Toms, J. (2008). Impact of oral assessment on physiotherapy students' learning in practice. *Physiotherapy Theory and Practice, 24(1),* 29-42.

Cohen, L., Manion, L. & Morrison, K. (2000) *Research Methods in Education* (5th edition). London: Routledge Farmer.

Coote, S., Alpine, L., Cassidy, C., Loughnane, M., McMahon, S., Meldrum, D., O'Connor, A. & O'Mahoney, M. (2007).The development and evaluation of a common assessment form for physiotherapy practice education in Ireland. *Physiotherapy Ireland, 28 (2),* 6-10.

Cowan, D. T., Norman, I. & Coopamah, V. (2005). Competence in nursing practice: A controversial concept – A focused review of literature. *Nurse Education Today, 25(5),* 355-362.

Cowburn, M., Nelson, P. & Williams, J. (2000). Assessment of Social Work students: Standpoint and strong objectivity. *Social Work Education, 19(6),* 627-637.

Crisp, B. R., Lister, P. G. & Dutton, K. (2006). Not just social work academics: The involvement of others in the assessment of social work students. *Social Work Education, 25(7),* 723-734.

Darke, P. Shanks, G. & Broadbent, M. (1998). Successfully completing case study research: combining rigour, relevance and pragmatism. *Information Systems Journal, 8,* 273-289.

Davis, M. H., Ponnamperuma, G. G. & Ker, J. S. (2009). Student perceptions of a portfolio education process. *Medical Education, 43,* 89-98.

Dearnley, C. A. & Meddings, F. S. (2007). Student self-assessment and its impact on learning - A pilot study. *Nurse Education Today, 27,* 333-340.

Duffy, K. (2004). *Failing students: a qualitative study of factors that influence the decisions regarding assessment of students' competence in practice.*, London: Nursing and Midwifery Council.

Dunworth, M. (2007). Joint assessment in inter-professional education: A consideration of some of the difficulties. *Social Work Education, 26 (4),* 414-422.

Elliot, T., Frazer, T. & Garrard, D. et al. (2005). Practice Learning and Assessment on BSc (Hons) Social Work: 'Service User Conversations'. *Social Work Education, 24(4),* 451-466.

Fisher, M., Callaghan, L., Snell, K. & Bellinger, A. (2010). An exploration of students' perceptions of practice assessment. *Nurse Education in Practice* [in progress].

Frankfort-Nachmias, C. & Nachmias, D. (1996). *Research Methods in the Social Sciences* (5th edition). London: Edward Arnold.

Ghaye, T. (2007). Is reflective practice ethical? (The case of the reflective portfolio). *Reflective practice, 8(2),* 151-162.

Hadfield, I., Murdoch, G., Smithers, J., Vaioleti, L. & Patterson, H. (2007). Is a professional portfolio, as a record of continued professional development, the most effective method to access a physiotherapist's competence? *New Zealand Journal of Physiotherapy, 35(2),* 72-83.

Hay, K. & O'Donoghue, K. (2009). Assessing social work field education: Towards standardising fieldwork assessment in New Zealand. *Social Work Education, 28(1),* 42-53.

Hobden, A. (2007). Continuing professional development for nurse prescribers. *Nurse Prescribing, 5(4),* 153-155.

Humphrey, C. (2007). Observing students' practice (through the looking glass and beyond). *Social Work Education, 26(7),* 723-736.

Jay, A. (2007). Students' perceptions of the OSCE: a valid assessment tool? *British Journal of Midwifery, 15(1),* 32-37.

Johnson, M. (2008). Grading in competence based qualifications – is it desirable and how might it affect validity? *Journal of Further and Higher Education, 32(2),* 173-184.

Kear, M. E. & Bear, M. (2007). Using portfolio evaluation for program outcome assessment. *Journal of Nurse Education, 46(3),* 109-114.

Kevin, J. (2006). Problems in the supervision and assessment of student nurses: Can clinical placement be improved? *Contemporary Nurse, 22(1),* 36-45.

Kneafsey, R. (2007). Developing skills in safe patient handling: Mentors' views about their role in supporting student nurses. *Nurse Education in Practice, 7(6),* 365-372.

Kneafsey, R. & Haigh, C. (2007). Learning safe patient handling skills: student nurse experiences of university and practice based education. *Nurse Education Today, 27,* 832-839.

Lauder, W. et al. (2008). Measuring competence, self-reported competence and self-efficacy in pre-registration students. *Nursing Standard, 22(20),* 35-43.

Lewis, C. E., Tillou, A., Yeh, M. W., Quach, C., Hiatt, J. R. & Hines, O. J. (2008). Web-based portfolios: A valuable tool for surgical education. *Journal of Surgical Research,* [article in press].

London, S. (2008). The assessment of clinical practice in osteopathic education: Is there a need to define a gold standard? *International Journal of Osteopathic Medicine, 11,* 132-136.

Luck, L. Jackson, D. & Usher, K.(2007). Case Study : a bridge across the paradigms *Nursing Inquiry, 13(2),* 103-109.

McCarthy, B. & Murphy, S. (2008). Assessing undergraduate nursing students in clinical practice: Do preceptors use assessment strategies? *Nurse Education Today, 28,* 301-313.

McCready, T. (2007). Portfolios and the assessment of competence in nursing: A literature review. *Journal of Nursing Studies, 44 (1),* 143-151.

McMullan, M. (2006). Students' perceptions on the use of portfolios in pre-registration nursing education: A questionnaire survey. *International Journal of Nursing Studies, 43,* 333-343.

McMullan, M. (2008). Using portfolios for clinical practice learning and assessment: The pre-registration nursing student's perspective. *Nurse Education Today, 28,* 873-879.

Miles, M. B. & Huberman, A. M. (1994). *Qualitative Data Analysis* (2nd edition). London: SAGE Publications.

Nairn, S., O'Brien, E., Traynor, V., Williams, G., Chapple, M. & Johnson, S. (2006). Student nurses' knowledge, skills and attitudes towards the use of portfolios in a school of nursing. *Issues in Clinical Nursing*, 1509-1520.

Norcini, J. J. (2005). Editorial: Where next with revalidation. *British Medical Journal, 330,* 1458-1459.

Payne, S., Field, D., Rolls, L., Hawkes, S. & Kerr, C. (2007). Case Study Research methods in end-of-life care reflections on three studies. *Journal of Advanced Nursing, 58(3),* 236-245.

Pirie, E. S. & Gray, M. A. (2007). Exploring the assessors' and nurses' experience of formal assessment of clinical competency in the administration of blood components. *Nurse Education in Practice, 7,* 215-227.

Ritchie, J. & Spencer, L. (1994). Qualitative data analysis for applied policy research. In A. Bryman & R.G. Burgess (Ed.), *Analyzing Qualitative Data* (173-193). London: Routledge.

Rushforth, H. E. (2007). Objective structured clinical examination (OSCE): review of the literature and implications for nursing education. *Nurse Education Today, 27(5),* 481-490.

Rushworth, H. (2008). Reflections on a study tour to explore history taking and physical assessment education. *Nurse Education in Practice, 8,* 31-40.

Rutkowski, K. (2007). Failure to fail: assessing nursing students' competence during practice placements. *Nursing Standard, 22(13),* 35-40.

Shapton, M. (2007). Failing to fail students in the caring professions: Is the assessment process failing the professions? *Journal of Practice Teaching and Learning, 7(2),* 39-54.

Sharpless, B. A. & Barber, J. P. (2009). A conceptual and empirical review of the meaning, measurement, development and teaching of intervention competence in clinical psychology. *Clinical Psychology Review, 29,* 47-56.

Smith, C. (1992). *Motivation and Personality: Handbook of Thematic Content Analysis.* Cambridge: Cambridge University Press.

Speers, J. (2008). Service user involvement in the assessment of a practice competency in mental health nursing – stakeholders' views and recommendations. *Nurse Education in Practice, 8,* 112-119.

Swigonski, M., Ward, K., Mama, R. S., Rodgers, J. & Belicose, R. (2006). An agenda for the future: Student portfolios in social work education. *Social Work Education, 25(8),* 812-823.

Vnuk, A., Owen, H. & Plummer, J. (2006). Assessing proficiency in adult basic life support: student and expert assessment and the impact of video recording. *Medical Teacher, 28(5),* 429-434.

Yin, R. K. (2003). *Case study research: design and methods* (3rd edition). London: SAGE Publications.

INDEX

A

academic settings, 33
accountability, 22, 32, 34, 36
accuracy, 3
anxiety, 12, 13, 17, 24
appointments, 7, 18
assessment tools, 19, 39, 44, 45
authenticity, 18
autonomy, 24, 29

B

benchmarking, 20
bias, 8
blame, 35
breakdown, 16

C

case study, 2, 5, 6, 8, 19, 52
clarity, 15, 20, 25
class, 29
clients, 13, 14, 22, 28, 33, 47
clinical assessment, 47
clinical examination, 51, 54
clinical psychology, 55
coding, 8
color, iv

communication skills, 19, 28, 29
community, 31
compilation, 3
confidentiality, 8, 13, 14
conflict, 28, 31, 33, 37
conflict of interest, 33
conflict resolution, 28
consensus, 15
consent, 8
consolidation, 34, 35
copyright, iv
creativity, 24
critical analysis, 29
cues, 4
curriculum, 15

D

damages, iv
data analysis, 54
data set, 45
detection, 33
direct observation, 18, 46
disappointment, 15
discomfort, 24
diversity, 2
drawing, 2
due process, 30

E

educational process, 17
educational settings, 6
electronic portfolios, 12
empathy, 28
ethics, 14
exclusion, 6
exercise, 14
experiences, 1, 2, 4, 6, 16, 17, 21, 25, 26, 30, 31, 32, 33, 34, 35, 36, 46, 51, 53
exploration, 52
exposure, 1

F

faith, 34
feedback, 3, 4, 13, 16, 17, 19, 20, 21, 25, 27, 29, 32, 33, 35, 44, 47
flexibility, 5
focus groups, 7, 42, 43
freedom, 2
freedom of expression, 2

G

general practitioner, 1
governance, 29
grades, 42
grading, 16, 20, 23, 43
group activities, 37
grouping, 11
guidance, 4, 15, 19, 21, 25, 26, 28, 46
guidelines, 26

H

health education, 39
honesty, vii, 15

I

individuality, 46
interpersonal skills, 28
intervention, 55
Ireland, 51, 52

L

leadership, 29
learners, 26
learning, vii, viii, 1, 2, 3, 4, 5, 12, 13, 15, 16, 17, 19, 22, 23, 24, 25, 27, 28, 29, 30, 31, 34, 35, 43, 45, 46, 47, 51, 52, 54
learning outcomes, 43, 51
learning process, 25, 47
longitudinal study, vii, 7, 15, 19

M

majority, 14, 28
management, 4
mental health, 55
mentor, 4, 15, 16, 20, 24, 27, 32, 33, 34, 36, 37
mentoring, 31
mentorship, 3, 22, 33, 51
messages, 20
methodology, vii, 5, 39, 44
modification, 7
motivation, 15, 23, 36

N

nerve, 19
New Zealand, 53
nurses, 53, 54
nursing, 31, 41, 51, 52, 54, 55

O

objectivity, 52

openness, 44
opportunities, 3, 27, 31, 32
OSCE, 3, 21, 51, 53, 54
osteopathy, 41
overlap, 27

P

parity, 20
peer assessment, 46
performance, 3, 16, 29
permission, iv
personal life, 37
pilot study, 52
politics, 24
portfolio, 3, 12, 13, 18, 20, 22, 23, 25, 26, 35, 46, 52, 53
positive relationship, 33
pragmatism, 52
pre-planning, 18
presentation skills, 20
prisoners, 18
professional development, 25, 34, 53
professionalism, vii, 32, 44
progress reports, 3
project, vii, 2, 4, 17

Q

qualifications, 53
questioning, 25

R

race, 29
reality, 14, 26
recognition, 22, 28, 33
recommendations, iv, 44, 45, 55
reflective practice, 53
reflexivity, 24
relevance, 52
reliability, vii, 2, 5, 8, 12, 15, 19, 23, 33, 45, 46, 47
resistance, 14

rights, iv

S

self-assessment, 3, 17, 52
self-awareness, 29
self-efficacy, 53
semi-structured interviews, 2, 7
smoothing, 35
social care, 1, 28
social change, 36
social sciences, 5
stakeholders, 2, 55
subjectivity, 15
supervision, 4, 22, 53
supervisor, 26
supervisors, 21
survey, 54
synthesis, vii, 8

T

testing, 37
thoughts, 17
time constraints, 21
training, 46
transcripts, 7, 8
triangulation, 23, 33
twist, 18, 36

U

United Kingdom, vii, 1, 2
updating, 36

V

validation, 8
variations, 26
video, 55

W

Webster, Daniel, 49

withdrawal, 6
workload, 20, 22
workplace, 1, 22, 25